About this book

Heal with Hormones is the third book I have published after the first book Heal with Detox and second book Heal with Diet. There are various case studies in this book which I hope to share, based on real life cases, on how balancing the hormones through the proper nutrition, nutraceuticals and hormone replacement therapies can help the body to heal. This book gathers evidence, based on data from journals and published papers, on the functions of different types of hormones in the male and female body and how they work together like the different instruments in an orchestra for the different metabolic functions of the body. It is also helpful for patients to have this as a guide to know which type of hormonal imbalances are causing their symptoms, do the appropriate testings, and work with a holistic or functional practitioner to rebalance their hormones.

In this book, I have also featured hormonal boosting recipes that are quick to prepare and provide a punch of nutrients to boost the hormones. Starting with the right diet and nutrients is the first step to winning the war against hormonal imbalance.

Hope you enjoy the reading as much as I enjoyed researching and writing this book.

Dedication

I dedicate this book to my parents who have taught me since young to always be humble and to follow my passion in whatever I do. Without them, I wouldn't be where I am today. I also dedicate this book to my dear husband Terry for always being my pillar of support and constantly encouraging me to pursue my passion in Functional Medicine. Finally, this book is dedicated to all my patients who are my best teachers. They have taught me that the body can heal itself when it is fed the right nutrients and exercise. Diseases and conditions can heal better when we treat them with a root cause approach. Special thanks and gratitude to all my teachers past and present and Dr Thomas Rau from Swiss Biomed Center who has shown me the world of biological medicine and is always so generous to share his knowledge with his students all over the world.

About the Author

Dr Ho See Yunn is a Family Physician with more than 15 years' experience. She is board certified in both Singapore and Hong Kong and received her specialization in Family Medicine from Singapore. Dr Ho holds a diploma from the New York Institute of Integrative Medicine in Integrative Health and Nutrition. She received her Advanced Fellowship in Functional and Nutritional medicine and peptide certification from the American Academy of Anti-ageing and Regenerative Medicine. In addition, Dr Ho received biological medicine training in the Swiss Biological Medicine Academy. Dr Ho is also trained and certified under Dr. Walsh's advanced nutrient therapy protocols that use personalized nutrient treatment strategies to treat patients with mood and behavioral disorders. Dr Ho believes in treating the patient holistically and finding the underlying root causes of disease. She takes a biochemical, nutritional and genetic approach in managing patients with chronic diseases.

"I have written this book with the hope that the content of this book will allow patients and practitioners to have a deeper understanding of the various hormones in the body and how they can use diet and nutritional supplementation or bioidentical hormone replacement therapies to rebalance their hormones and achieve a better hormonal harmony in the body. It may be confusing to navigate the many supplements and hormone protocols in the market but it is my hope that this book will provide a roadmap to navigate you on a journey to achieve better hormone balance and optimize the function of the body." - Dr Ho See Yunn

Disclaimer

This book is accumulated from hours of research but is still a work in progress and cannot be considered as a diagnostic or treatment manual. As much as I have tried to present the information in this book as accurately as possible, data changes rather fast and I can only hope to update the information in this book to keep it as current as possible. Though every effort has been made to ensure the accuracy of the information in this book, it is not meant to provide medical advice as that can only come from your own treating physician. The material contained in this book is not intended to be a substitute for proper medical advice from one's own physician or other healthcare providers. It simply reflects the latest thoughts and trends in this field and from my own personal experiences. I would also like to put a disclaimer that I do not have any financial ties to any supplement or pharmaceutical company or laboratory in the process of writing this book. The author of this book shall not be liable for any loss, injury, or damage arising from any information in this book.

Acknowledgements

I would like to thank God for guiding me to be at a unique position where I am – not just a conventional trained doctor, but also a doctor that has been trained in Functional Medicine and in the Swiss Biological method of healing. I would also like to thank my parents for being always supportive of me and enabling me to always pursue my dreams to be a doctor since I was a child. I am forever grateful to my mum and dad for teaching me the bible and I dedicate this book to my dad whose medical condition led me into functional medicine to treat patients from the root cause of their problems.

Last but not least, I would like to thank my husband Terry for always encouraging me to pursue my passion in Functional medicine and getting my training and certification despite having to juggle my role as a busy clinician and a mum of three (while writing this book the third one came along). He is always supportive of me to continue studying and helping to take care of the family while I continue to pursue my passion. This book would not see its light without my husband constantly encouraging me. Thank you to my three kids whom God has blessed me with and they are always a guiding light for me, spurring me on to be a good human being

Contents

Disclaimer

Chapter I

Hormones and Menopause

Symptoms of low estrogen - Hot flushes and mood swings

Case study:

Ms K is a pleasant Korean lady who saw me previously for chronic fatigue issues but we lost touch for almost a year due to her travels. Her work is often very intense and stressful which also led to her suffering from low mood and anxiety which she is taking medication for. This year she came to see me in February with a different kind of symptoms - hot flushes. That was what raised my suspicion that she was going into menopause. Her period has totally stopped since June last year and she only had some spotting in December. In October, she had a full body check up done in Korea and was found to have low estradiol level with raised FSH and LH. Her hot flushes were preventing her from falling asleep and when she does fall asleep, she tends to wake up around 3-4am every night and couldn't fall back asleep. Because of her lack of sleep, she was feeling low in mood and energy. She tried using alcohol to help her to sleep and ended up drinking more than she should. Her libido has also fallen which is also aggravated by her having vaginal dryness and pain. To add to her misery, she was also having central weight gain. No matter how hard she is exercising, she couldn't seem to shed the weight from her middle. Her other symptoms include having brain fogginess and difficulty in remembering things especially affecting her work in the past 1 year.She just couldn't concentrate at work.

We did the hormone panel for her and the findings confirmed her menopause. Her estradiol level has reached menopausal level at <5pg/mL, progesterone was <0.8ng/mL, testosterone was <11.5ng/dL and cortisol level was 1.4ug/dL. That explained why she was having such severe hot flushes, waking up at night and also low libido! Her cortisol level was so low because of her many years of stressful working life which could have led to her adrenal fatigue. And when cortisol is so low, it could further create hormonal havoc.

For her brain forgetfulness besides low estrogen, I also tested her pregnenolone level which was also very low at 12 ng/dL. That explains why her brain couldn't function properly and she was having these short term forgetfulness.

When she came for review, she finally came to realize that the deficiency of her hormones are the root cause of all the symptoms she had been experiencing the past year. We discussed the benefits and cons of bioidentical hormone therapy *and because of her severe symptoms, she decided to go ahead with the treatment. She was also given adrenal complex to help boost her low cortisol so that it could better balance her other sex hormones. Testosterone replacement therapy was also started to help improve her libido and energy.*

About 2 months later when Ms K came for her next review, she had felt much better and the hot flushes were almost gone with the estrogen replacement. The progesterone replacement has helped her to sleep better and deeper and she was waking up refreshed and feeling more energy. With the extra estrogen, her brain function and memory were also improving and she could concentrate better at work and she no longer felt so much anxiety or low mood that she used to be having before the treatment. She was also able to keep her weight down from 56kg a few months ago while she was in Korea, to the current weight of 53Kg.

Low estrogen

Estrogen is the female hormone that makes a woman have feminine characteristics. It is responsible for maintaining the health of the female uterus, vagina and urethral tissues. It is also responsible for maintaining a healthy brain function by exerting its effect on the prefrontal cortex and hippocampus which is responsible for verbal memory. Estrogen is also responsible for increasing the enzymes needed for the synthesis of acetylcholine responsible for memory function in the brain.

Most of the estrogen produced during the reproductive years is 80% made up of estradiol (E2), 10% is made up of estriol (E3) mainly produced in pregnancy, and 10% is made up of estrone (E1) which is the main estrogen during menopause. Estrogen is a jack of many hats and its multiple functions include:

Mood

For women suffering from mood swings due to low estrogen, you would like to know that estrogen is responsible for regulating the amount of serotonin, the "Feel-good hormone" and serotonin receptors in the brain. Many menopausal women with low estrogen often complain of unexplained low mood, sometimes even becoming suicidal.

Thermoregulatory effects

Perimenopausal or menopausal women with declining estrogen will experience severe hot flushes and night sweats which may affect their sleep.

Sexual characteristics

Estrogen is responsible for maintaining the moisture and sensitivity of the vagina and without estrogen, women usually feel like sex is "the last thought on their mind". The vaginal tissues become dry and painful during intercourse. Some women who experience laxity in their vaginal and urethral tissues due to a lack of estrogen will also start experiencing worsening urinary or stress incontinence.

Heart and bone protection

Estrogen does have its benefits in terms of heart and bone protection during the perimenopausal years. That is why after menopause, women are at an increased risk of heart disease and osteoporosis. Estrogen prevents the buildup of inflammation in the coronary vessels and maintains healthy cholesterol levels. For bone protection, estrogen promotes the activity of osteoblasts which helps in bone metabolism to improve bone density.

During perimenopause usually from the age of 45 years old, estrogen levels will start to decline. The level of estrogen during perimenopause is usually 20-30% higher than menopausal levels but they fluctuate more widely. Especially in women who are facing high stress, the high cortisol can cause the level of estrogen to fluctuate more widely which can lead to symptoms like hot flushes appearing earlier during perimenopause. It is common to hear of women complaining of hot flushes and mood swings appearing during the perimenopausal years. Vaginal dryness and pain can also appear due to falling estrogen levels leading to thinning and inflammation of the vaginal tissues. This can lead to disinterest in sex and also urinary incontinence issues.

Ways to manage low estrogen

1) Diet and lifestyle changes
   - Increase the intake of phytoestrogen in the diet. Eat organic whole soy made tofu, miso soup or

natto, and non GMO soymilk. All these plant based phytoestrogens can help to reduce symptoms of estrogen deficiency.(3)
- Avoid too much caffeine in the diet as to much caffeine and coffee has been shown to lower estradiol level in women.(4)
- Increase the intake of sesame seeds, sesame oil and flaxseeds in your meals. These seeds contain lignans (similar structure to phytoestrogens) which act on estrogen receptors to help ease the symptoms of hot flushes etc. The flaxseeds also offer an additional fiber to the diet which help maintain good bowel movements.
- Pomegranate or pomegranate seed oil has been shown to help ease the symptoms of hot flushes and other symptoms of menopause. (5)

2) Nutraceuticals
- Take Vitamin E supplement about 400IU/day. Studies have shown that taking Vitamin E at dosage of 400 IU/day helps reduce hot flushes and increase the blood supply to the vaginal wall.
- Magnesium has been shown to help reduce symptoms of anxiety and hot flushes during menopause.
- Black cohash at 40g-80g / day has been found in various studies to help reduce menopausal symptoms. A 2010 study has shown that black

cohash helps reduce night sweats and hot flushes in menopausal women.(6) However, be careful of black cohash as high doses can cause liver issues.

- Evening Primrose Oil, an important plant phytoestrogen, has been shown to be effective in reducing night sweat and hot flushes. (7)
- Red ginseng has been found to help to improve energy, mood and sense of well-being in postmenopausal women.Ginseng acts of estrogen receptors to exert estrogenic effects.(8)

3) Bioidentical hormone replacement
- Bioidentical hormones are favored over synthetic hormones as they are the exact molecular structure to the hormones that your body makes. Synthetic hormones have a different chemical structure than the natural hormones in the body. It is important to work with a trusted practitioner who is experienced in BHRT to also discuss if there are any risk factors that may contraindicate the use of BHRT.
- A strong indication to start Bioidentical estrogen therapy earlier will be:
  - Mood changes like depression or anxiety which comes on during perimenopause due to a lack of estrogen. Instead of turning to antidepressants, these women should first be treated with estrogen. In

one study, women respond better to stress after menopause when they have estrogen replacement via a patch. (1)

- ○ Severe hot flushes that affect daily activities and affect sleep.
- ○ Brain fog issues that affect daily activities like forgetfulness and difficulty concentrating.
- ○ Insomnia that doesn't improve with supplements.
- ○ Headaches or migraines that come on due to a lack of estrogen.
- ○ Vaginal dryness may be alleviated with topical estrogen creams.

- Any woman who starts on estrogen replacement must always counterbalance the estrogen with progesterone to prevent endometrial tissue build-up. Some other benefits of bioidentical progesterone include:

- ○ Improving deep sleep, no waking up in the middle of the night.
- ○ It is a natural GABA neuroinhibitor which helps to calm the woman down and reduce anxiety.
- ○ Less fluid retention, improves estrogen progesterone ratio balance.

***

Menopause Symptom

Symptoms of low progesterone - Mood swing and anxiety, insomnia

---

Ms J is a pleasant lady who previously saw me for gut bloating issues. This time when she came to see me, she was 55yr of age and presenting with a different set of symptoms - that of poor sleep and severe anxiety. She used to sleep very well but in recent months, started waking up in the middle of the night. Melatonin that used to work for her doesn't help her sleep now. In addition to that she was feeling more anxiety than she used to. Her only son had just gone off to university and she was feeling much more anxiety symptoms than she used to have. On questioning, the past year her period had become more irregular. It came in April, May, June then stretched to once every 1-2 months August, September, November. Because of her poor sleep, she is also experiencing more fatigue and brain fogginess with lack of concentration. Her hormonal blood test revealed that her estradiol level had declined to 13pg/mL and progesterone level to <0.8ng/mL which is near menopausal level. For her waking up at night and anxiety symptoms, it is most likely due to the low progesterone level and she was started on micronized progesterone tablets 100mg daily at bedtime to help with her sleep issues. After about 2 weeks taking the progesterone and with the menopause supplement support, she was feeling better and was able to sleep throughout the night. Her anxiety was also greatly reduced and she was feeling in better control of her symptoms. She was also started on magnesium and evening primrose oil to reduce inflammation and her symptoms of anxiety. She was advised on a diet to increase intake of good clean fats and *phytoestrogens which also helped to ease her symptoms of hot flushes. Overall after a few months of rebalancing her hormones, she was feeling back to normal and was able to return to her daily function without the emotional rollercoaster she was feeling before.*

Low Progesterone

Throughout the fertile years of a woman, the ovaries are responsible for producing healthy levels of estrogen, progesterone and testosterone.

It is important to have a good balance ratio of estrogen to progesterone for the woman to feel most optimal. Although they follow a rhythmic pattern throughout the menstrual cycle, they need to maintain the delicate balance like two sides of a seesaw to make the woman feel most optimal.

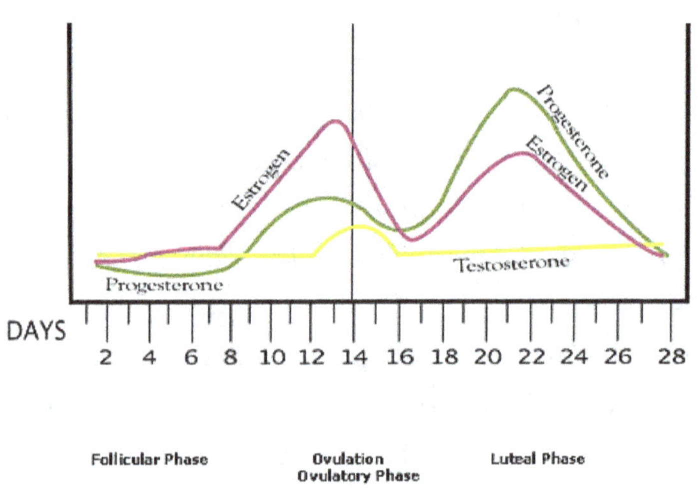

From the diagram above, progesterone level usually comes up during the second part of the cycle called the luteal phase. They are responsible for building the endometrial lining to prepare the womb for fertility and implantation. That is why low progesterone levels can lead to fertility issues. Also, when the progesterone level is low, it does not balance the effects of estrogen and as a result it leads to a condition called estrogen dominance. The unopposed estrogen is like a horse without a rein - leading to more inflammation, cysts or fibroids formation, endometriosis, or PMS issues like migraines, poor sleep and period pains etc. Excess estrogen can also lead to abnormal uterine bleeding and even stimulate endometrial cells to become malignant.

The role of progesterone besides helping to balance estrogen, is also to work as a neuroinhibitor to help with reducing anxiety and helps maintain a good deep sleep at night. Progesterone works on the GABA receptors and makes the woman feel more relaxed and calm.

Ideally, if you measure your progesterone level during day 19-21 of your cycle, you would want the level of serum progesterone to be about 10-25ng/mL and the ratio of progesterone to estrogen to be about 100-400 to be in a balanced state.

For women with poor sleep due to low progesterone levels, I would recommend seeing the doctor to prescribe 100mg to 200mg of micronized progesterone to help restore good deep sleep, rather than just turning to sleeping pills. Usually for my patients with poor sleep onset during perimenopause or menopause, prescribing them the progesterone would usually help them to sleep deeper and feel more calm and relaxed.

What causes PMS? - the broken dance between estrogen and progesterone

PMS is a sign of imbalance progesterone to estrogen ratio leading to symptoms like heightened anxiety, poor sleep, hormonal headaches and mood swings. This points to an issue between progesterone, the GABA receptors and serotonin. PMS has been postulated to be due to "progesterone resistance", and the GABA receptors are not receptive to progesterone - like a key which doesn't fit into the lock. This creates a hormonal havoc during the luteal phase, causing mood swings or even low mood. Sometimes giving a bit of 5HTP to lift the serotonin level may help alleviate the mood swings during this period.

Stress and the Pregnenolone Steal

Most people know progesterone to be produced in the ovaries. However, a small amount of progesterone is also produced in the adrenal glands. The adrenal glands first produce this pre-hormone called pregnenolone which then produces progesterone and goes on to produce cortisol. In stressed women where cortisol is very high to produce a constant "fight or flight" response, the progesterone goes to produce more cortisol which is the termed the pregnenolone steal. To make matters worse, the high cortisol also sits on the progesterone receptors like an unwelcome guest, vying with progesterone for its seat at the table. With not much progesterone left and with no receptors to bind to, the woman starts to feel the effect of low progesterone - heightened anxiety, restlessness and poor sleep. As progesterone is also a diuretic, the woman also suffers from fluid retention due to the lack of progesterone. That is why a lot of stressed young women nowadays have problems trying to have a baby, this is due to a lack of progesterone due to the "pregnenolone steal". Without progesterone to maintain the endometrial lining for implantation, the chance of fertility diminishes.

Ways to increase progesterone

1) Diet and lifestyle changes
   - Reduce stress to reduce cortisol
   - Reduce caffeine intake. This is because caffeine raises cortisol which vies with progesterone for the receptors causing symptoms of low progesterone.
   - Eat more good fats like avocados, nuts and seeds like pumpkin seeds, sunflower seeds, sesame seeds. These good fats are the raw materials for helping your body produce progesterone.

2) Nutraceuticals
   - Vitamin C at about 1g/day. This has been shown to raise progesterone level during the luteal phase. (1)

- Chasteberry (Vitex agnus-castus). Take this at a dose of 500-1000 mg/day. This herb helps stimulate the pituitary to release luteinizing hormone (LH) which raises progesterone. In women with fertility issues, chaste berry has been shown to improve progesterone levels and fertility rates. (2)

3) Bioidentical hormone replacement
  - In women who are perimenopausal or menopausal where the ovaries are no longer responsive to chasteberry stimulation, consider the use of bioidentical hormones either via progesterone creams or tablets. These bioidentical progesterone replacements are molecularly similar to your natural progesterone. For insomnia symptoms, I would usually recommend oral micronized progesterone as it passes the blood brain barrier to help symptoms of insomnia. Micronized progesterone in 100mg or 200mg dosage usually helps my patients sleep well through the night.
  - Avoid synthetic Progestins that have been shown to increase risk of breast cancer, depression, weight gain and blood clots.
  - For progesterone creams, they are helpful for hot flushes. Start from the dosage of 20mg, 40mg or 60mg.

Chapter 2

Estrogen Dominance and Related Gynecological Issues

Case study: Estrogen dominance and endometriosis

Ms J is a pleasant 32yr old lady and was referred by her friend to come see me. She was diagnosed with having endometriotic cysts on both sides of her ovaries measuring about 3 cm each. She wanted to come see me to see what we can do on a functional approach to help her endometriosis even though her gynecologist simply says to observe and have a "wait and see" approach as the cysts were still small.

We discussed the functional approach to treat endometriosis through first making a change in her diet to a more anti-inflammatory diet and to remove hormone exposures through meat and dairy products. I advised her to cut down gluten, sugars and dairy in her diet to reduce the inflammation that is associated with endometriosis. We also discussed increasing omega 3 in her diet and supplementation to help reduce inflammation.

We checked her hormone level on day 21 of her cycle and found that her progesterone estrogen ratio on day 21 was low, indicating that she was estrogen dominant. She was advised to increase fiber and cruciferous vegetables in her diet to help her body to detoxify the excess estrogen in her body. I also started her on a DIM supplement which is made up of broccoli extract to enhance estrogen detoxification. In addition to that, she was started on omega 3s, curcumin and vitamin D to help reduce inflammation associated with endometriosis.

Ms J was very diligent and followed a clean diet that is both anti-inflammatory and enhancing detoxification. She also took the supplements religiously. We followed this regime and after about 6 months when she followed up with her gynecologist, her cysts were getting smaller and till date, they have become undetectable. During the process, Ms J also got pregnant as her cysts were getting smaller and she was more hormonally balanced. She was glad that not only did her endometriotic cysts disappear, she was also able to achieve hormonal nirvana and even delivered a healthy adorable baby.

***

Estrogen dominance

Estrogen is required to maintain the feminine characteristics of a woman. However, it is crucial to maintain the delicate dance between estrogen and progesterone as too much estrogen or too little progesterone to balance the estrogen can mean estrogen is dancing with a non existent partner and this can lead to a condition called Estrogen Dominance.

Some of the important functions of estrogen include:

- Giving the woman the feminine characteristics like hips and breast, and also maintaining the skin turgor and volume.
- Estrogen in its well balanced state helps to regulate serotonin, the happy hormone, to help lift the mood.
- Estrogen builds the endometrial lining in the first half of the cycle to prepare for conception, if there is any egg for implantation.

Estrogen, like the creative artist, is always stimulating, but it needs the progesterone, the discipline master to hold it in its rein. Estrogen and progesterone need to be in a balanced state and we usually test the level of the progesterone and estrogen on day 21 of the cycle. The ratio of progesterone to estrogen to be a good range is between 100-400. If the ratio is less than that, it signifies that there is progesterone deficiency or estrogen excess. Excess estrogen is like a bull without a rein, and it can wreck hormonal havoc. Some symptoms of estrogen dominance include:

- Breast tenderness
- Water retention
- Pelvic tenderness and period pains
- Extreme mood swings, anxiety
- Headaches or migraines
- Poor sleep with frequent waking up at night
- It can even lead to gynecological issues like endometriosis, ovarian and breast cysts
- Weight gain

What causes excess estrogen?

During the reproductive years from age 12 to 45, estrogen is made mainly in the ovaries with 80% of that consisting of estradiol E2, 10% is estrone E1 and 10% is estriol E3.

During menopause, the ovaries starts to shut down the production and estrogen becomes mainly produced from our fat cells. During the menopausal years, the estrogen made in the body is mainly estrone E1. E1 is the bad one amongst the 3 charlie angels and is the one we want less of and to detoxify it more from the body.

Estrogen is detoxified in the liver via 2 phases: phase I which is the hydroxylation phase and phase II which is the conjugation phase. During phase I hydroxylation, estradiol and estrone are metabolized into 2hydroxy estradiol, 2hydroxyestrone, 16hydroxyestrone or 4 hydroxyestrone. 2 hydroxyestradiol and 2 hydroxyestrone are the protective metabolites whereas the 4hydroxy and 16hydroxy estrone are the bad guys which can be carcinogenic. Studies have found that a higher ratio of 2:16 hydroestrone is associated with a lower breast cancer profile.

Then during phase II liver detoxification a process called conjugation occurs whereby these metabolites are conjugated with a chemical group called glucuronic acid making the metabolites more water soluble to enhance their excretion via the bile, the stools and the urine.

Some women with genetic issues with their detoxification genes in phase I of the pathway may upregulate the toxic estrogen metabolites more than their body can handle and these may form DNA adducts and become carcinogenic, triggering breast, endometrial or cervical cancer in women. Women with genetic issues with their phase II detoxification genes may have problems conjugating these toxic metabolites out of the body and hence these excess estrogen accumulates in the body.

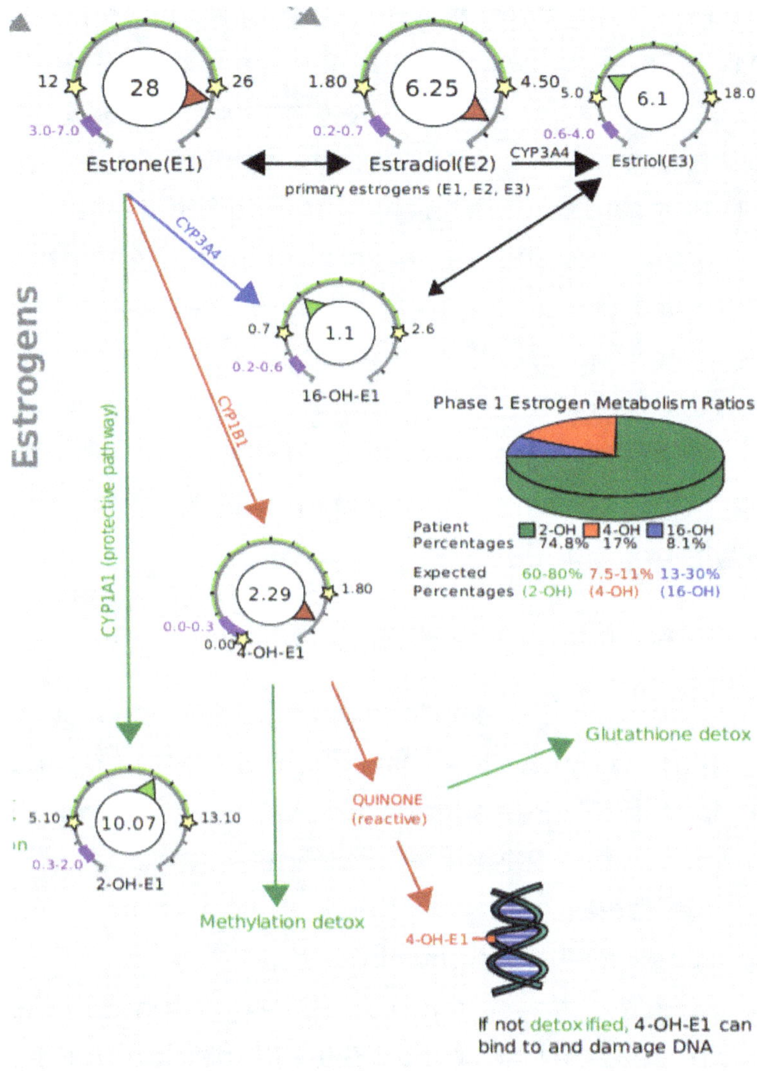

(adapted from the DUTCH test)

So excess estrogen can accumulate due to problems with detoxifying it and excreting it from the body. Excess estrogen could also be from external sources of estrogen that we are exposed to in our food and environment. Xenoestrogens are chemicals in our environment usually from products we use everyday that can mimic estrogen. These include plastics, BPA, phthalates, flame retardants, fragrances put into our shampoos and soaps, and many more of these organic pollutants. These xenoestrogens are also called endocrine disruptors and they can bind to estrogen receptors on breast or endometrial cells causing cellular proliferation and carcinogenesis. These xenoestrogens are like uninvited guests to a party, taking up the seats of those invited guests and leaving a trail of destruction when they leave. What is scary is that these xenoestrogens are found insidiously in our everyday products including deodorants, sunscreens, makeup, can food lining, plastic food wraps making it hard for us to identify or avoid.

Ways we can avoid these xenoestrogens in our daily lives:

- Reduce or stop eating foods out of canned foods as these cans usually have BPA lining which can leak into our foods.
- Instead of drinking from plastic water bottles, drink from glass water bottles or BPA-free water bottles.
- Use fragrance free soaps and shampoos that are made from natural organic ingredients.
- Avoid microwaving food using plastic containers or plastic covers as the high heat can cause the plastic phthalates to leak into the foods.

- Try to eat organic produce as many of the foods nowadays contain pesticides and herbicides.

Ways to reduce excess estrogen and improve estrogen detoxification

- Diet and lifestyle changes
    - Eat organic, grass fed meats that are hormone free to reduce exposure to hormones in the meats that you eat.
    - Increase the intake of cruciferous vegetables including broccoli, brussel sprouts, cauliflower etc as these vegetables increase the phase II liver detoxification to remove the estrogen metabolites from the body.
    - Eat a high fiber diet as the fiber helps to bind the excess estrogen to excrete them in the stools.
    - Reduce exposure to dairy products like cow's milk, cheese and yogurt as these dairy products contain extra hormones from the female cow.

- Nutraceuticals
    - Take DIM supplements at 100mg 2 times a day to enhance liver detoxification of the estrogen metabolites.
    - For patients with endometriosis and ovarian cysts caused by estrogen dominance, take omega 3s 1gm daily and curcumin 500mg 2 times a day to reduce inflammation associated with estrogen dominance.

Chapter 3

Hormones and Weight Gain

Case study: Ms SW

Ms S is a pleasant 50 year old lady originally from Australia but has been in Hong Kong for about 20 years. She works as a teacher and faces high stress in her job. She presented as a new patient to me in June 2022. At that time, she was highly stressed after getting retrenched from her previous job and was also suffering from low mood due to her mum passing away at the beginning of the year. To make matters worse, her period had stopped around October of 2021 and she was having symptoms of menopause like hot flushes and frequent waking up at night. This has also made her more anxious. But her main symptom that really bothered her was her unexplained weight gain. She had previously always been slim in her 40s but since the beginning of last year, she had gained 8 Kg even though she has always eaten healthy and exercised vigorously 5 times a week doing hiking, biking, running and swimming. She was at her wits end as she had tried everything and couldn't lose weight. She was finding it so difficult to put on muscle even though she exercises almost daily.

The hormone panel done for Ms SW showed that she is likely suffering from hypothyroidism which explained her weight gain. Her TSH level was >4uIU/mL and she has low levels of fT3 and fT4. Her DHEA level was also low at 122 ug/dL and testosterone level was low at 15ng/dL. That explained why she was also feeling so fatigued and was having difficulty putting on muscles despite her exercises. Although her estrogen level was maintained high at >200pg/mL, her progesterone level was non-existent at <0.8ng/mL which puts her in an estrogen dominance mode. This can cause her to feel extreme mood swings, anxiety and also cause the waking up at night. We discussed the next steps which is to start the thyroid medication to improve her thyroid function and metabolism. She was also started on DHEA 10mg tablets to help improve her fatigue. She was given DIM tablets to help reduce her high estrogen and progesterone tablets 100mg at bedtime was started to help her have a better sleep through the night and reduce her fluid retention. She was also advised on a clean keto protein diet to help with her weight management.

She came back a month later elated that she had lost 6KG just making the changes in her diet and starting on the thyroid medication and supplements to improve her metabolism and hormone balance. She felt less fluid retention, leaner and was able to fit into her previous clothes again. She was so happy with her progress and was feeling so much better in her mood and her anxiety had vanished along with her weight. Miss SW successful weight management is a testament that just balancing and controlling hormonal imbalance could help improve the body's metabolism and enhance weight loss.

***

Thyroid hormones and weight

In recent years, many people are jumping onto the bandwagon using peptides like semaglutide injections for weight loss. However, a better strategy for maintaining weight would be to dig into the root cause - usually hormone imbalance - why there is weight gain in the first place and correct the underlying hormone imbalance.

Thyroid gland is a master gland situated in the front of the neck that is responsible for maintaining the metabolism of the body. This explains why people who suffer from hypothyroidism can suffer from weight gain and other symptoms like fatigue, cold intolerance, low mood, hair loss and dry skin. Thyroid hormone also controls the body's reaction to other hormones like cortisol and estrogen. However, for patients with weight gain, many of them don't get their thyroid checked, or rather, the doctor will check just the TSH and tell them that their thyroid is normal. They end up suffering for many years from low thyroid feeling sluggish, having unexplained weight gain, loss of hair thinking that these symptoms are all normal parts of aging but they are not. Hypothyroidism is especially common amongst women after their forties. Statistics show that more than 20 percent of those women above their forties are taking thyroid medications (this number may be even more just that many cases of hypothyroidism are left unchecked).

Many of these patients with weight issues like Ms SW can improve their metabolism and get their weight coming down when they address the root cause and correct their hypothyroidism with the appropriate thyroid medications. The latest data has shown that treating even subclinical hypothyroidism can improve outcomes in the patients. Sometimes even with a normal TSH level, the patient may have low triiodothyronine (fT3) due to endocrine disruptors that vie with the thyroid hormones for the thyroid receptors. Correcting this low fT3 can help improve the symptoms of fatigue and weight gain for these patients.

Case study 2: Ms DS

Ms DS is a 49 yr old pleasant South African lady and she has been seeing me mainly for the symptoms of menopause. Her symptoms of mainly hot flushes were controlled by the estrogen replacement. She was also having a lot of anxiety symptoms due to her highly stressful job and waking up frequently in the middle of the night. These symptoms improved with the oral progesterone tablets 200mg given to her at bedtime every night. Another major complaint for Ms DS was that of difficulty shedding her weight. In recent years, she has gained weight to her current weight of 74kg. She wanted to get back to her previous weight of 70kg but despite her best efforts to eat a clean keto healthy diet and exercising 3 times a week, she was finding her difficult to shed her extra kilos. During one of her visits, she was having so much anxiety associated with palpitations and shortness of breath that I ordered a full thyroid panel for her. The test results revealed that her Triiodothyronine (T3) was low at 1.93pg/mL, her fT4 was 0.80ng/dL and her TSH was 2.05uU/mL. Due to her low fT3, she was started on thyroid medications to improve her fT3 and TSH level which will in turn help her to improve her symptoms of fatigue, her metabolism and weight.

A month later, I bumped into Ms DS on the street and she was looking radiant and happy and leaner. She told me that the thyroid treatment really did wonders for her and it was the missing piece that improved all her symptoms. She was feeling much better and all her palpitations were gone. She also felt leaner and was able to lose some weight. This case really highlighted to me how correcting the thyroid, even a single T3 could actually make a huge difference to the patient's symptoms and weight.

Testing the thyroid function

- The good range of TSH is between 0.3 - 2.5mIU/L.
- T4 produced by the thyroid gland is the inactive form of the thyroid hormone. It needs to be converted to the active form T3 to make the body more metabolically active. T3 has a greater impact on how much energy the body produces.
- In normal situations when the body is healthy, T4 is mostly converted to T3, but only a small portion gets converted to reverseT3, the useless form of T3. In some situations when the body is stressed or during caloric restriction, the body produces more reverse T3 and the

body becomes more thyroid resistant and suffers from hypothyroid symptoms despite a normal TSH level. As such, do not rely on just a normal TSH or T4 to deduce a "normal thyroid". One study has found that people who have been found to have low serum T3 and high reverse T3 actually have poorer physical performances than those with normal T3 level.

- In patients with low T3, adding a small dose of T3 in the treatment may help improve the symptoms by a lot. Keep fT3 levels optimal between 2.5-3.4ng/dL.
- Women during perimenopause or menopause are more likely to suffer from thyroid issues, so don't forget to check the thyroid panel as part of the overall hormone assessment. About 25% of women over 60yrs old develop thyroid antibodies which may attack their thyroid gland and cause symptoms of hypothyroidism.

Ways to manage low thyroid function

1) Diet and lifestyle changes
   - Ensure adequate stress control by incorporating stress reduction techniques as high stress can affect the cortisol which can disrupt thyroid function.
   - Ensure adequate dietary intake of iodine which is the raw material for production of thyroid hormones. Iodine is found in

food sources like seaweed, kelp and iodized salt.

○ Avoid goitrigens by avoiding eating raw broccoli, kale and brussel sprouts as these goitrogens may lead to decreased thyroid function.

2) Nutraceuticals

○ Zinc is important for the healthy conversion of T4 to T3, reducing the conversion to reverseT3. Keep zinc dosage about 15mg per day. Take this with 2mg of copper to maintain a good zinc copper balance for optimal thyroid function.

○ Take selenium supplement at recommended dose of 200mcg per day. Selenium is an antioxidant that helps protect the thyroid from oxidative stress and also reduce the immune hyperactivity from thyroid antibodies.

○ Ensure adequate iron level as adequate iron level is important to maintain optimal thyroid function. Low iron reduces the function of the enzyme thyroid peroxidase which helps to convert T4 to active T3. Keep ferritin level in the healthy range between 70-90.

○ Get adequate vitamin D as vitamin D deficiency can lead to autoimmune thyroid disorders.

3) Bioidentical hormone replacement

○ Some patients feel symptomatically better and prefer to start with glandular which are natural desiccated thyroid which have both T3 and T4 which are more physiologically similar to our body's thyroid hormones.

○ Patients usually feel better on natural desiccated thyroid than synthetic T4 thyroxine as desiccated thyroid contains 80% T4 and 20% T3 with some T1 and T2 - and this combination is more physiologically similar to the body's thyroid gland. Always start with the lowest dose and work the dosage upwards based on the optimal thyroid level range.

○ Add T3 as needed if the fT3 is low. There are 2 forms - Cytomel and compounded T3. Always start with the lowest dose 5 mcg and be careful with T3 as it is four times more potent than T4 and may induce anxiety and heart palpitations.

○ It usually takes 4-6 weeks for the level of thyroid hormone to stabilize.

***

Polycystic Ovarian Syndrome

Case study: Ms AK

Ms A is a pleasant 19yr old lady who came to see me with her parents with the main complaints of acne skin and unexplained weight gain. She had been having acne issues since she was a teenager but in the recent 1-2 years, it has worsened into an inflammatory state with redness and scarring. The acne flare-ups are usually worse the week before her periods. She also had been struggling with weight issues for a long time but this year, she tried a gluten free diet and lost 4-5 Kg in weight. But she finds that her weight yoyos according to her diet and once she goes off the diet, she will easily put back on the weight again. Her period had always been irregular ever since menarche, but last year she tried acupuncture to help the hormone imbalance and since then, her period had become regular again. Last year she consulted with a gynecologist who did an ultrasound and found that she had polycystic ovaries. Her mood has been low and she often suffers from anxiety due to her weight issues.

Her hormone panel blood test revealed that she was having high estrogen 266 pg/ml compared to progesterone 10.6ng/mL and her testosterone was on a higher end of the range at 40.6ng/dL. This higher testosterone was causing her skin to break out with cystic acne along her jawline and on her forehead. The progesterone estrogen ratio was 40 indicating that she was in estrogen dominance which can account for symptoms of fluid retention, PMS mood swings and also worsening of her acne before her periods. She was also found to have insulin on the higher range at 9.9 uU/mL which is an early sign of insulin resistance causing her weight gain.

This was how her cystic acne looks due to her high testosterone hormone and estrogen dominance.

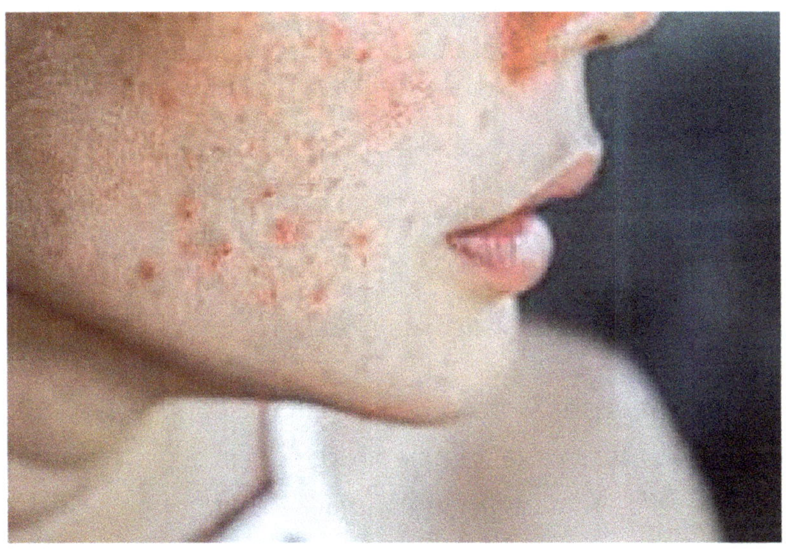

We worked on reducing her testosterone with spironolactone and she was also given DIM supplements to reduce the high estrogen stimulation and vitex to boost her progesterone to improve the progesterone estrogen ratio so as to improve her mood and sleep. As she was struggling to lose weight, she was started on the peptide Saxenda to improve her insulin resistance and help accelerate her weight loss.

We discussed her diet to switch to an anti-inflammatory diet high in Omega 3, low in gluten, dairy and sugars which can *cause inflammation. Instead, she was encouraged to eat more fruits and vegetables for Vitamin C and antioxidants to help her skin.*

Ms AK came back for review and felt that her acne has improved greatly with the change in diet and improving her hormone balance which made a difference in reducing her inflammatory cystic acne on her face. She also lost a few pounds and gained more confidence in her appearance. She was also having better mood and sleep and less PMS symptoms due to better hormone control.

***

Polycystic Ovarian Syndrome (PCOS)

PCOS affects 20% of women and it is a condition whereby the androgens in the female body goes on an overdrive causing excessive hair growth and acne eruptions on the skin. There are various ways of characterizing PCOS but some of the diagnostic criteria includes finding cysts on the ovaries, insulin resistance and high testosterone level. However, not all PCOS patients fulfill all these criteria and hence many females with PCOS go undiagnosed.

Females need some testosterone in their body to help with their libido, muscle growth and generally to feel more confident and strong. However when androgens are in excess, for example during PCOS, testosterone can be converted by an enzyme called aromatase into estrogen. This excess estrogen can further make it difficult to lose weight. Too much testosterone in the female can also lead to mood issues like irritability, depression and anxiety

High testosterone also gets converted to dihydrotestosterone (DHT) which can cause male pattern hair loss in women. So besides having acne, women with PCOS also suffer from thinning locks especially around the temples.

Besides high androgen, another hormone that gets dysfunctional in PCOS is Insulin. Many PCOS patients suffer from Insulin Resistance - which is the state whereby the pancreas becomes insensitive to Insulin causing blood glucose to rise. High glucose in the body leads to more inflammation, weight gain and more oxidative stress to the cells. It also leads to a higher incidence of diabetes and heart disease. High insulin also leads to a higher androgen level by lowering sex hormone binding globulin leading to higher free testosterone levels in the body. High insulin also leads to a downward spiral of more inflammation in the body by triggering interleukins and cytokines.

For PCOS patients, it is good to ask your doctor to test the following hormone levels for you:

- Serum testosterone level
- Serum estrogen to progesterone ratio to look for estrogen dominance
- Check DHT level is experiencing hair loss
- Fasting glucose and Insulin level

Many PCOS patients also typically develop many small cysts on their ovaries which looks like "a string of pearls' ' on the ultrasound. These cysts are non functional and don't go into ovulation and hence there is a lower chance to get pregnant causing subfertility in PCOS patients.

Ways to manage a high androgen level and inflammation associated with PCOS

1) Diet and lifestyle changes
   - PCOS is an inflammatory condition. It is advisable to have an anti-inflammatory diet by reducing gluten intake as gluten can create silent inflammation especially in those with gluten sensitivity.
   - Reduce dairy in the diet especially cow's milk products including cheese and yoghurt. Dairy contains hormones from the mother cow and also cow's proteins that can create inflammation in sensitive individuals.
   - Reduce high glycemic index foods or foods high in sugars and carbohydrates as these foods can lead to high glucose levels especially in PCOS patients with insulin resistance. High sugar levels create inflammation in the body.
   - Reduce intake of vegetable oils like sunflower or canola oil which are high in

omega 6. Avoid fried foods as these are usually fried with palm oil or vegetable oils which can create more inflammation. Instead opt for foods which are higher in omega 3s. Use healthy oils like olive oil or avocado oil. Eat more omega 3 rich foods like fatty salmon or chia and flax seeds.

- ○ Eat foods which are high in antioxidants like blueberries, strawberries, blackberries etc. Colorful fruits and vegetables are high in phytonutrients like lycopene, beta carotene which help to reduce oxidative stress on the cells.
- ○ Eat meats that are hormone-free, preferable organic or grass-fed beef and hormone free chicken. Meats that contain hormones injected into them can further cause hormone disruption ina the PCOS patients with estrogen dominance.
- ○ Eating foods high in zinc as zinc is crucial for maintaining healthy menstruation and ovulation. Zinc intake also helps in skin repair during acne outbreaks. It helps in reducing skin inflammation, aiding in repair of inflammatory acne and reducing scarring. Examples of foods high in zinc include beans, nuts and seeds.

○ Stress reduction techniques are important to help reduce the high stress and cortisol in patients with PCOS.

○ Acupuncture is helpful in regulating the hormone imbalance and improving ovulation and fertility in patients with PCOS.

2) Nutraceuticals

○ Take berberine, cinnamon and chromium supplements that help with metabolizing sugars and help sensitize the pancreas to insulin so as to help reduce insulin resistance. Take chromium picolinate at a dosage of 200-1000mcg per day.

○ Inositol is a sugar structure made in the body and found in foods. There are 2 forms D-chiro-inositol and myo-inositol. Inositol plays a role in insulin signaling and helps improve insulin resistance and improve fertility in PCOS patients (9). Dosage is about 2-4gm/day.

○ Saw Palmetto helps reduce high androgens in the PCOS patients and reduce the conversion of testosterone to DHT which can cause hair thinning and hair loss. Dosage is about 160 mg/day.

○ Take omega 3s 1-2g/day and bioactive curcumin 500mg-1gm/day to help reduce the inflammation associated with the condition of PCOS.

O Taking vitamin D at a dosage of 2000-5000 IU/day helps balance the immune system and reduce the inflammation and metabolic disturbance in the body. Vitamin D replacement also helps improve the mood of patients suffering from depression in PCOS.

Chapter 4

Hormones and Fertility

Low Progesterone

Case Study: Ms KC

Ms KC is a 36 yr old young lady who was referred by a fellow practitioner to see me to work on her fertility issues. She has good past health with no other major health issues. She has been trying for a baby with her husband for more than a year but with no success. A year ago, she did a fertility screening and was told by her doctor that everything was normal. Her uterine structure was also found to be normal.

Upon questioning, her periods are usually regular but come once every 38-40 days and last 5-7 days each time. Her period cycle is longer than a normal female cycle which is usually 28-30 days. Her PMS symptoms are mainly that of breast pain the week before her period.

She also complained of having sleep issues and not sleeping well at night with frequent waking up.

From her symptoms, of PMS breast pains with frequent waking up at night, I had the suspicion that her progesterone is low and ordered the Dutch Cycle Mapping Test to look at her levels of progesterone during ovulation and the luteal phase and this was her result:

Estrogen (E) patterns can be seen below in green. Progesterone (Pg) patterns can be seen below in purple. Normal ranges are within the gray dashed lines. See page 2 for more information.

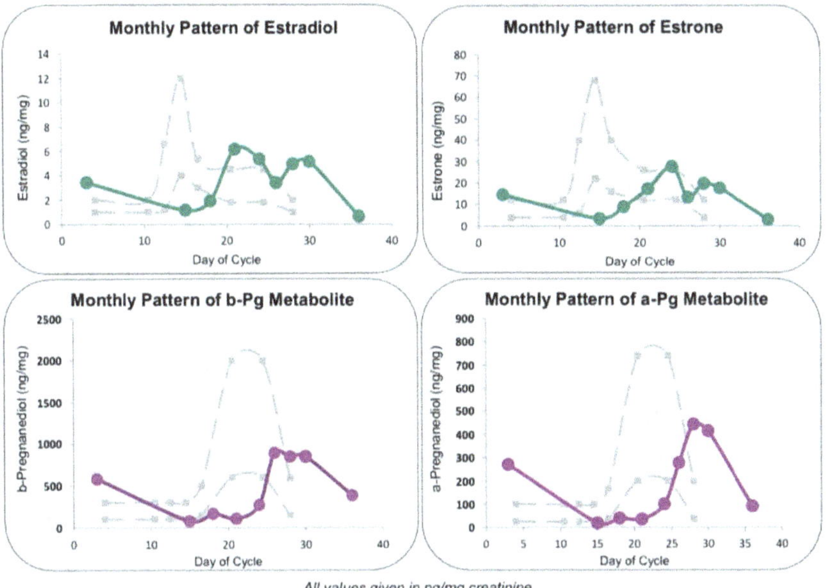

All values given in ng/mg creatinine

From her result, it can be seen that she is suspected of having a luteal phase defect and ovulation is later than the typical day 10-14. This is also followed by a progesterone peak that is less than ideal. A low progesterone level can lead to infertility as there won't be adequate endometrial lining for the implantation of the fetus to occur.

For Ms KC, I started her on Vitex (chasteberry) 750mg per day and advised her to time her ovulation to be later around day 20 rather than the usual day 10-14 of the cycle.

Low progesterone and subfertility

During each menstrual cycle, estrogen and progesterone work together in a clockwork manner. In the first phase of the cycle, estrogen starts building up which also causes the uterine lining to build up and become thicker. Then ovulation occurs whereby the follicles secrete progesterone which starts to build up the next phase of the cycle - the luteal phase. During this phase progesterone rises and stops the endometrium from becoming thicker and to prepare the endometrial lining for the fertilized egg for implantation. There must be sufficient progesterone during this phase to ensure the change of the endometrial lining to mature and to prepare for the egg to implant if there is any which leads to pregnancy. If conception does not occur, progesterone level starts to drop which leads to the shedding of the endometrial lining called menstruation. If implantation occurs, progesterone levels continue to rise to stabilize the fertilized egg and support the developing fetus.

The second part of the cycle is known as the luteal phase and the term "luteal phase defect" means that the ovaries are not producing enough progesterone in the second half of the cycle and hence the endometrial lining is not stable enough for implantation and breaks down.

Some laboratory criteria for diagnosing "luteal phase defect" is that you may have low progesterone on day 19-21 of the menstrual cycle or when you do the hormone cycle mapping, you will find that the progesterone does not achieve the desired "peak" during day 21 but instead peaks at a lower level at a later part of the cycle. This luteal phase defect occurs in 10 percent of women with infertility or 35 percent of women with miscarriages. However with infertility or miscarriages, there are other factors that must be addressed including structural problems with the uterus, genetic deficiencies etc.

Ways to manage infertility associated with low progesterone

1) Diet and lifestyle changes
    - Eat a diet higher in good fats as having good fats help in hormone production. Foods that high in clean fats include avocado, nuts like almonds, walnuts, and seeds including pumpkin seeds, sunflower seeds etc.
    - Do the seed cycling regime which is eating seeds like flax seeds and pumpkin seeds before ovulation and after ovulation in the luteal phase, eat seeds like sunflower seeds and sesame seeds to boost progesterone production.
    - Manage stress as high cortisol can vie with progesterone for the receptors and

also lead to the pregnenolone steal with reduced progesterone production. Doing daily stress reduction techniques like breathing and meditation exercises helps in keeping cortisol levels at a healthy level.

- ○ Avoid drinking too much coffee as caffeine can disrupt the cortisol level which affects progesterone. Instead switch to more herbal teas like rooibos tea or decaffeinated green tea.

2) Nutraceuticals

- ○ For premenopausal women, take vitex (chaste berry) at 750 mg to 1 gm per day. This helps to stimulate the production of Luteinizing hormone to stimulate the ovaries to produce more progesterone. Take chasteberry for at least 2-3 months to see a beneficial effect on improving progesterone and also regulating the menstrual cycle. In a study of women with low progesterone and fertility issues, the participants who have been taking chasteberry were found to have a higher rate of fertility. (10)
- ○ Taking Vitamin C 1gm/day has been shown to help low progesterone and

improve those with luteal phase defect. (11)

3) Bioidentical hormones
    ○ For women who have reached menopause, the ovaries are less able to produce progesterone and they may need external progesterone either oral progesterone or progesterone creams.
    ○ Some fertility doctors may prescribe oral progesterone tablets at 100-200 mg daily to bring up the progesterone faster during the luteal phase. Avoid taking synthetic progestins as it can worsen mood issues and has been shown to increase risk of blood clots and heart disease.

Chapter 5

Testosterone - is it only for males?

I) Testosterone for females

Many women are surprised when told that testosterone plays a role in their bodies. Isn't testosterone a male hormone, why do I need that too? In fact, testosterone does play an important role in the orchestra of hormones in the woman's body besides estrogen and progesterone. In women, testosterone helps in maintaining a healthy libido (sex drive), promoting lean body muscle mass, and helps to upkeep the memory and mood. The quantity produced in the woman is 250mcg per day whereas males produce about twenty to forty times more than that.

In males, testosterone is produced mainly in the testes and adrenal glands whereas in women, testosterone is produced mainly in the ovaries and the adrenal glands. The highest level of testosterone occurs in women in their twenties but the level declines every year. Many women patients I see often have very low testosterone levels by the time they reach their forties and almost nonexistent by the time they are menopausal. It is not surprising then to hear women complaining of disinterest in sex by the time they reach their forties due to their low testosterone level. This low level of testosterone is due to the lower adrenal gland production. It is interesting to know that 50% of testosterone production comes from conversion from DHEA in the skin and fat tissues, 25% from adrenal gland production and 25% from ovaries production.

Another common complaint amongst female patients who have low testosterone is that of central weight gain and difficulty losing weight no matter how hard they are exercising or watching their diet. Low testosterone leads to lower lean body muscle mass and instead, more adipose tissues and accumulation of fat especially around the intra abdominal region. One study published by the Journal of Clinical Endocrinology and Metabolism showed that women who were given testosterone replacement therapy lost double the amount of fat and gained more muscle mass which helped them lose weight compared to those given a placebo.

The benefits of testosterone in females include:
- Improve libido
- Increasing muscle mass, strength and tone
- Helps in losing weight especially the abdominal area
- Better mood
- Better memory
- Improved energy and motivation
- Improved bone strength and density
- Maintaining healthy skin and hair

II) Testosterone in males - do males benefit from testosterone replacement therapy ?

Case study:

Mr M is a pleasant 40yr old English gentleman who came to see me recommended by one of his gym friends. He had been battling with his divorce issues for the last 2 years and had experienced low mood and anxiety. He also has the complaint of low libido and erectile dysfunction which he needs to take Viagra for and this frequently gives him a headache. The erectile issues could likely also have contributed to his marriage issues. His job isn't too stressful but the main stress he is facing now is from his divorce. The past 2 years, he had gained 10kg likely from the stress eating but since late last year he has switched to a protein diet and since lost about 5kg of weight. He used to be a professional rugby player and knew how to eat well for his nutrition. He currently eats a more protein diet consisting of eggs, meat proteins and salad. He exercises intensely going to the gym 4 times a week doing resistance exercises and 2 times a week of HIT training. We did a health screening hormone panel for him and found that his testosterone level was suboptimal at 480 ng/dL (optimal levels for males will be 600-1000 ng/dL). We discussed his diet to incorporate more healthy fats in his diet to help his hormone production and continue his HIT training which would also help boost his testosterone production. He was also advised on stress reduction techniques and given supplements to manage his stress cortisol to avoid the stress eating. For his suboptimal testosterone and his current symptoms of low libido, low mood, weight gain and poor sleep, we discussed how the testosterone replacement therapy may boost his testosterone level and help improve his symptoms. Since he already has two children and fertility is not a consideration for him, he decided to give Sustanon a try and to come in 2 weekly for the injections. He started feeling an improvement a month into the injection and upon review 3 months later, he was happy that he had noticed an improvement in his low mood and anxiety and was feeling more energized. He had also been sleeping better since starting the hormone injections. His libido has also improved and he no longer has problems with erectile dysfunction. To add to his delight, he had also lost another 5-6 Kg of weight since starting the testosterone injection. He was motivated to continue his diet of high protein but also incorporating good clean fats in his diet to help boost his hormone production.

***

Male hypogonadism, often known as "Low T," is a disorder in which the body produces insufficient amounts of hormones due to problems with the brain, pituitary gland, or testicles. Testosterone replacement treatment, also known as androgen replacement therapy, is licensed to treat this condition. To aid with weariness, erectile dysfunction, and lack of sex drive, men utilize patches, gels, tablets, injections, or creams with testosterone.

Testosterone therapy is used to treat male hypogonadism, also called "low testosterone" or "Low T." This is a condition in which the body doesn't make enough hormones because of an issue involving the brain, pituitary gland, or testicles. Hypogonadism can be treated with a variety of prescription testosterone products. Different testosterone products include gels, injectable solutions, patches, pills, and pellets that are put under the skin.

Once a person starts testosterone therapy, they usually have to take it for the rest of their lives. The patient's hormone levels will be checked every six months. Depending on the patient, the checkups may be more often.

- Each year, U.S. men spend $2 billion on testosterone.
- In 2014, four times as many men as in 2000 were using testosterone products.
- In 2013, testosterone therapy was used to treat 2.3 million people in the U.S.
- In 2011, almost one out of every 25 men in their 60s took testosterone.
- From 1988 to 2011, the amount of testosterone sold with a prescription went from $18 million to $1.6 billion.

Causes of testosterone deficiency and decline that starts around the 30s

Testosterone levels vary widely from one man to another and even from day to day. The decrease in testosterone levels is often gradual. However, it may be sharp in some men. A drop in testosterone can be caused by a number of circumstances, including:

- **Aging:** After age 30, men's testosterone levels gradually decline. This decline accelerates after age 40 when men lose about 1% of their testosterone yearly.
- **Illness:** Certain chronic illnesses, such as diabetes and kidney disease, are associated with decreased testosterone production.
- **Injury:** Injury to the testicles can cause a sudden drop in testosterone levels.
- **Medications:** Some medications, such as corticosteroids and opiates, can decrease testosterone production.
- **Obesity:** Men who are obese have lower levels of testosterone than men of healthy weight.
- **Stress:** Severe stress, such as that experienced during a major illness or injury, can decrease testosterone production.

Ways to boost testosterone levels in males

1) *Diet and lifestyle changes*

There are a few **testosterone booster foods**
- **Oysters:** Oysters are a great source of zinc essential for testosterone production.
- **Beef:** Beef is rich in zinc, iron, and magnesium. It's also an excellent protein source, essential for muscle growth.

Doing HIIT (High intensity Interval Training) exercise has been found to boost testosterone production in men. One study found that men doing interval training consisting of 90 seconds of intense treadmill running interspersed with 90-second recovery periods boosted free T levels more significantly than simply running for 45 minutes straight. (12)

Reduce stress level by doing stress reduction exercises as high cortisol from high stress can reduce androgen production.

Avoid exposures to external xenoestrogen like BPA and phthalates as they are endocrine disruptors that can affect the testosterone receptors.

2) Nutraceuticals that help boost testosterone

Testosterone supplements help testosterone Some of the nutrients that help to produce and maintain **increase testosterone** include:

- **Vitamin D:** Research has shown that vitamin D is crucial for testosterone production. One study found that men who were deficient in vitamin D had lower testosterone levels than those who weren't.
- **Zinc:** Zinc is another nutrient that's essential for testosterone production. It's found in foods like oysters, beef, and pumpkin seeds.

- **Magnesium:** Magnesium plays a role in over 300 biochemical reactions in the body and has been shown to boost testosterone levels.
- **Fenugreek:** Fenugreek is an herb used for centuries in traditional medicine. It's thought to increase testosterone levels by stimulating the production of luteinizing hormone, which regulates testosterone production.

3) Bioidentical hormone replacement

Testosterone Products Come in Many Forms

Testosterone can be given as an injection, a patch, a gel for the skin, or a cream. It can also be given as a solution on the armpit, patch, or buccal system on the upper gum or inner cheek.

Even though you need a doctor's prescription for many testosterone products, some drug stores, and health food stores sell them without a prescription. Some of these products also say they are made from natural ingredients.

Gels (Androgel)

Testosterone gel is a prescription drug on a man's shoulders, upper arms, and stomach, depending on the brand. Testosterone gel can get out of your body and into other people's, which can cause serious health problems. To avoid this:

1. Put testosterone gel on skin that will be covered by clothing and is clean, dry, and whole.
2. When you're done, wash your hands with soap and water.
3. Once the gel has dried, cover the area with clothing and keep it protected until you have passed the area well or showered.

Getting shots:

Sustanon and Nebido injections are available in the market for testosterone replacement therapy.

Sustanon:

It is a pale yellow colour injection containing testosterone as an active ingredient. Usually people get one shot every 2 weeks of Sustanon. It is used in people suffering from low testosterone for testosterone replacement therapy. It treats various conditions caused by low levels of testosterone in adult males. Sustanon is available in the market in 250 mg packing and injected into muscles by only registered doctors or nurses.

Nebido:

Nebido is a clear yellowish oily solution used as an injection for long-term testosterone replacement therapy. It is available on the market in 1000 mg/4 vials injected once in 3 months. It is injected into your muscles and stored in your body for a long time. It is released from the body gradually and maintains testosterone levels in the body.

Transdermal patches (Androderm)

Testosterone transdermal patches, like Androderm, are skin patches that deliver testosterone. Patches work best when they are put on every night around the same time and left on for 24 hours. Testosterone patches should always be worn until they need to be changed. Every 24 hours, you should change your Androderm patch. Before putting on the new patch, the old one should be taken off. You should put a patch on a different spot each night and wait at least seven days before using the same spot again.

Two kinds of hormones are used to make testosterone products:

- Bioidentical Hormones

Bioidentical hormones are in AndroGel and several other products. In a lab, scientists make hormones that are chemically the same as the hormones that the body produces on its own. In theory, this will have less of an effect on other things.

- Synthetic Hormones

Synthetic hormones are made from chemicals that have been changed from their original forms, so they do not match the hormones the body makes. Most of the time, these kinds of drugs have more side effects.

Alternatives to maintain fertility

Sperm production decreased in people undergoing TRT. Because the external source of testosterone suppresses the body's production of testosterone and ultimately sperm production. Some alternatives like HCG (human chorionic gonadotropin) injection and clomiphene are used for men who still would like to maintain fertility while undergoing TRT. This therapy maintains sperm production.

Chapter 6

Diet for Enhancing Hormonal Health

Hormone Boosting Nutrients

The key to balancing your hormones starts, not from using bioidentical hormones, but from having a good nutrition and lifestyle. "What? You mean what I eat can help balance my hormones?" This is the usual response I get from my patients whenI talk about diet and nutrition with them. Usually, when they see a doctor for their period problems, they will usually be prescribed oral contraceptives to suppress all their hormones or hormone replacement therapy (HRT) to replace their hormones. However, from all the patients I have managed for their menopausal or hormonal issues, I find that those patients who have the best results are those who change their diet and lifestyle which leads to a better hormone balance.

Here are some tips for the Do's and Don'ts for foods that help balance your hormones.

Do have more of these foods:

- Eat more antioxidants and phytonutrients in your diet. These foods help reduce inflammation associated with hormonal imbalance and reduce oxidative stress on the cells.
- Eat foods that are high in Omega 3s to help reduce inflammation associated with hormonal decline.
- Eat clean, lean and hormone free meats. These proteins contain tryptophans which help to boost serotonin to improve mood swings in patients with hormonal imbalance.
- Eat good fats. Good fats help in production of hormones. They also help to make one feel fuller and not have food cravings which helps maintain a healthy weight.
- Eat fiber daily with each meal. Fiber helps in detoxification of estrogen from the body through the stools.
- Eat organic and hormone free produce.
- Eat a greater amount of cruciferous vegetables like broccoli, cauliflower and cabbage. This group of vegetables contain sulforaphane which help in detoxification of estrogen by the liver to excrete it out from the body.
- Eat more spices like turmeric, rosemary, thyme etc as these helps to reduce inflammation and provide a higher antioxidant level to the body.

	Foods to eat	**Examples of foods**
For improving cellular health	Foods high in antioxidants and phytonutrients	<ul><li>Blueberries, strawberries, cherries</li><li>Color vegetables like bell peppers, tomatoes, carrots, beetroots etc.</li></ul>
To help reduce inflammation	Foods high in Omega 3	<ul><li>Fatty fish like salmon, cod fish 2 times a week</li><li>Chia or flax seeds are high in Omega 3</li></ul>
For mood boosting	Eat clean, lean proteins to help boost serotonin level	Organic chicken, turkey, fish, grass-fed beef
For hormone production	Eat good fats	Including avocado, nuts like almond and walnuts, seeds

		including sunflower, sesame seeds, flax seeds and pumpkin seeds
For estrogen detoxification	Eat fiber with each meal	Fiber comes from eating fruits and vegetables with each meal, psyllium husk
For estrogen detoxification	Eat a greater amount of cruciferous vegetables	Include broccoli, cauliflower, cabbage, brussel sprouts

Foods to avoid

- Avoid dairy products, especially cow's milk. Cow's milk contains hormones which can disrupt the body's hormones.
- Avoid a high sugar or high carb diet. High sugars can lead to greater inflammation and also lead to mood swings and energy slumps. HIgh sugar and carbohydrates can also lead to weight gain.
- Avoid cooking with vegetable oils like canola or sunflower oil and avoid foods fried in palm oil as these oils can create more inflammation in the body. Instead cook with olive or avocado oils.

- Avoid eating from plastic containers or drinking from plastic bottles as these can contain BPA which can lead to hormone disruption.

7 Day Detox Diet for Hormonal Reset

For my patients who are having hormonal issues, be it weight gain from menopause of sluggishness from thyroid problems, it is good to start with a 7 Day Detox and Hormone Reset diet to improve the alkalinity of the body and enhance liver detoxification of excess hormones which helps to reduce inflammation of the body.

This diet consists of :

- A 16 hour fast to enhance autophagy of the body to clear dead cells and improve the body's metabolism.
- A green juice cleanse in the morning.
- A lunch high in protein and amino acids to enhance the liver detoxification process.
- A vegetable broth for dinner at night to improve alkalinity of the body.
- Higher intake of cruciferous vegetables to enhance phase II liver detoxification.

Example of a 7 Day Detox Diet Plan

Meal Plan	Monday	Tuesday	Wednesday	Thursday	Friday	Saturday	Sunday
16 HR FAST	skip breakfast	skip breakfast	skip breakfast	skip breakfast	skip breakfast	skip breakfast	skip breakfast
BREAK FAST 12PM	Green Juice	Green Juice	Green Juice	Green Juice	Green Juice	Green Juice	Green Juice
LUNCH	Tumeric Tofu salad	Poached chicken with green salad	Alaskan salmon with bean salad	Asian minced chicken with lettuce wrap	Broccoli and mushroom stirfry	Baked tumeric coated cauliflower rice	Sunday roast chicken with broccoli salad
SNACK	Handful of nuts	blueberry chia pudding	carrot sticks with almond butter	edamame hummus	protein bar	nuts	blueberry chia pudding
DINNER	Vegetable mineral broth, rainbow salad	Broccoli zucchini soup	Cauliflower rice with couscous, raisins and walnuts	Vegetable mineral broth with couscous tomatoes and red onion salad	Broccoli, garlic and mushroom stirfry	Steam brussel sprouts with sesame and tahini dressings	Baked tumeric coated cauliflower rice
DRINKS	Green tea	Green tea	Green tea	Green tea	Green tea	Green tea	Green tea

Clean-Keto-16 Diet to enhance hormone balance, improve metabolism and weight

Going into a ketogenic diet is an effective way to lose weight fast as when our bodies are deprived of carbohydrates, the body does not have anything else to burn but fats, hence it goes into a "fat-burn" mode. Besides burning fat, the body also feels more energized due to the greater energy expenditure and faster metabolism. Ketones also help provide more energy to the brain.

A ketogenic diet also helps optimize sugar and insulin levels. High insulin from the constant supply of glucose can lead to fat deposition so when insulin levels go down, fat-burning rate goes up.

Another benefit of ketosis is when there are good fats and proteins, the level of hunger hormones like Ghrelin and Leptin balances and leads to less hunger pangs.

Alkalinity in the diet helps reduce inflammation and reduces cortisol which is responsible for belly fat. Alkaline foods also help support detoxification of toxins out of the body. Alkaline rich foods also help preserve muscle and bone density as it retains minerals in our body.

The traditional ketogenic diet is high in fats (saturated), moderate proteins and low in carbs. This helps burn fat efficiently but can make the body very acidic and inflamed, thus causing symptoms of fatigue, gut disturbances which are known as the "keto flu".

This Clean Keto Diet focuses on a ketogenic diet but also on nutrients that makes the body more alkaline thus reducing inflammation while turning the body into a fat burn mode.

The principles of this diet are:

- restricting your carbs to less than 40 gm a day.
- Eat "clean-keto" foods - whole, unprocessed foods high in fiber, low in carbs but packed with nutrients. Examples include lots of green leafy vegetables, nuts and seeds, avocados, coconut oil, ghee.
- Avoid "dirty-keto" foods like bacon, pork, high fat beef, processed cheese, dairy milk.

- Focus on good fats like olive oil, olives, avocados, coconut oil, nuts, seeds.
- Have moderate amounts of organic lean proteins like grass-fed beef, organic free range poultry, wild-caught fish, vegetarian protein like tofu, tempeh. Proteins are natural metabolism boosters.
- Add lots of alkalizing vegetables including leafy greens like spinach, lettuce, kale, chard, beet greens, collard greens, and cruciferous vegetables including broccoli, Brussel sprouts, cauliflower. These are low in carbs but high in nutrients, vitamins and antioxidants.
- Add in intermittent fasting (IF) of about 16 hours everyday to enhance autophagy (the clearing of dead cells) and boost metabolism for weight loss.
- Observing a 80/20 ratio of alkali to acidic foods - consume 80% vegetables and 20% acidic foods like proteins and healthy fats.
- Test your urine for alkalinity and ketones throughout the 14 day diet as that gives information on how you are burning fat.

Recipes for enhancing hormone balance

These recipes are created with considerations to support these organs for hormone balance:

Adrenal glands

The Adrenal gland is the master gland in the body like the maestro of the orchestra. It controls the proper function of other hormones in the body. Cortisol is produced from the adrenal gland which helps regulate metabolism, immune and stress response of the body. Too much cortisol can lead to adrenal stress and too low cortisol can lead to adrenal fatigue. The nutrients that help maintain healthy adrenals include Omega 3, Vitamins B5, B6, and B12, Vitamin C and Magnesium. Healthy fats containing Omega 3s are found in fatty fish like salmon and codfish and B vitamins are found in red meat or organ meats and dark green vegetables like spinach and kale. Healthy fats found in avocados, olive oil, nuts and seeds help in the production of hormones from the adrenal glands.

Thyroid Gland

The thyroid gland controls the metabolism of the body and is responsible for maintaining proper heart rate, body weight, body temperature, normal menstrual cycles etc. Too much thyroid hormones can lead to palpitations and anxiety, too little can cause weight gain, fatigue, irregular menstrual cycles and hair loss. The nutrients that help maintain a healthy thyroid gland include iodine found in seafood and seaweed, selenium found in brazil nuts and eggs, and iron found in red meat and dark green vegetables.

Liver Support

Many people forget about the liver when it comes to the topic of hormones, but the liver is the major organ that helps to detoxify excess hormones like estrogen from the body through the phase I and phase II detoxification. Without a healthy liver to help in detoxification, the liver can't burn fat well and this leads to weight gain and sluggishness. For maintaining a healthy liver, include nutrients like indole-3-carbinol which are found in cruciferous vegetables like broccoli, cauliflower, cabbage, brussel sprouts etc. Foods high in antioxidants like beetroots, blueberries, colorful bell peppers and pomegranate help protect the liver cells from damage.

Gut health support

Maintaining proper gut health helps in maintaining good bowel movements which is important for the detoxification of hormones and keeping the immune system healthy. The gut wall is also lined with serotonin receptors and "a healthy gut keeps a healthy mind". Foods high in fiber and prebiotics help support healthy gut bacteria. Fermented foods like Kimchi and sauerkraut are high in probiotics to help in fighting off nasty bacteria. Legumes contain fiber and are also resistant starches which helps maintain a stable blood sugar level.

Recipes

Recipe 1) Breakfast Paleo Avocado Almond Pancakes

Avocadoes pack a punch of healthy vitamins and minerals and most importantly, provide good clean fats that enhance hormone production. For making pancakes, they provide moisture and act as a binding agent to bind the ingredients together. Use a ripe avocado in this recipe for easy blending.

This recipe uses gluten free flour and coconut oil for making the pancakes.

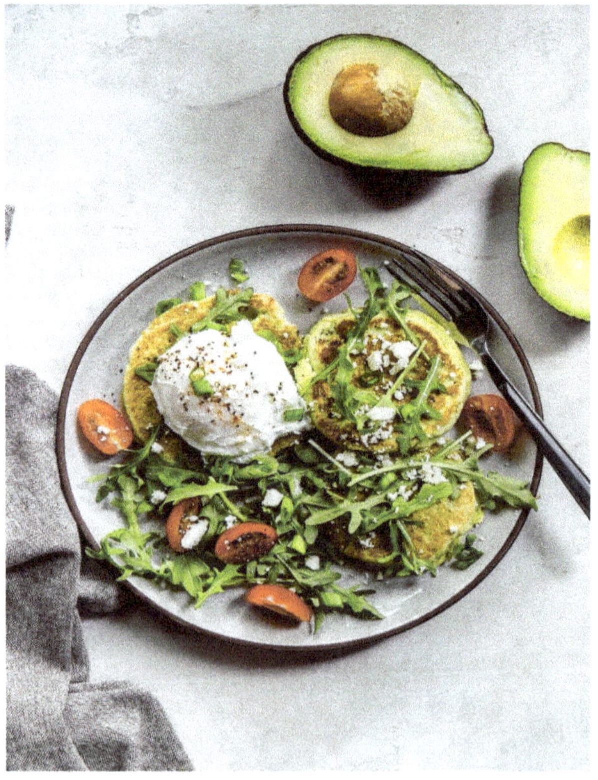

Prep time: 15min
Cook time:20 min
Servings: 10 pancakes

Ingredients:

- ❖ 2 eggs
- ❖ 1 ripe organic avocado peeled and deseeded.
- ❖ ¾ cup almond milk or coconut milk
- ❖ 2 cups fine almond flour
- ❖ ¼ cup gluten free flour
- ❖ 1 tsp baking powder
- ❖ Pinch of salt

Directions:

1. Combine all ingredients in a blender. Blend until completely smooth. Batter will be very thick - add a bit more almond milk if the batter is too thick.
2. Heat a non-stick frying pan over medium-low heat and add enough coconut oil to coat the surface.
3. Once the pan is completely hot, measure ¼ cup of pancake batter and pour onto the hot surface. Usea spatula to spread the batter into a circular shape.
4. Cook 2 minutes on one side of the pancake until it begins to firm up. Carefully flip and cook for another 2 minutes, or until the pancake is cooked through. Repeat these steps for the remaining batter.
5. Serve pancakes with a poached egg on top or for a sweet pancake, drizzle with organic maple syrup.
6. Enjoy!

Recipe 2) Hormone and Omega 3 Enhancing Avocado, Salmon and Egg Bake

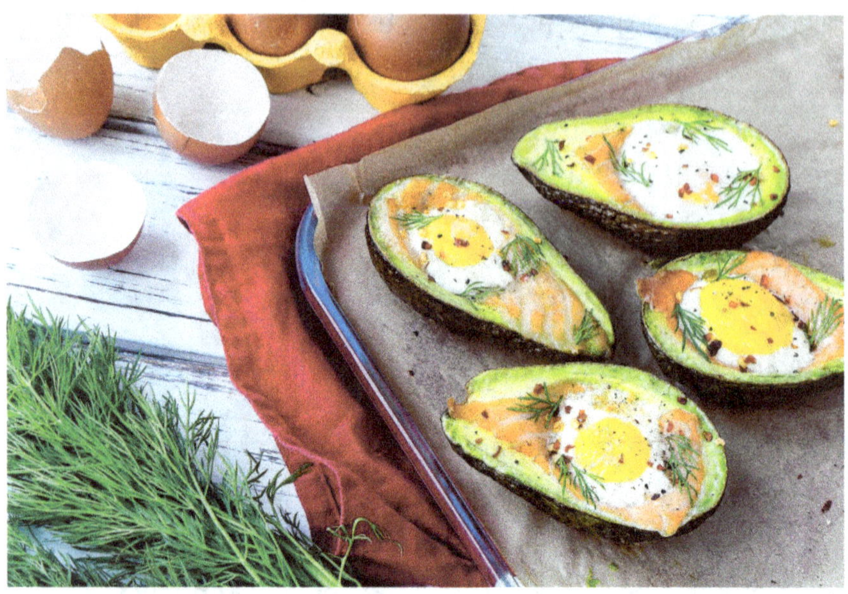

This recipe is great for enhancing hormone balance with the good fats from avocado and the omega 3 from the salmon helps reduce inflammation. Eggs provide a good source of choline for maintaining healthy cell membranes in the brain and liver.

Servings: 8
Prep time: 10 min
Cooking time: 15 min

Ingredients:

- ❖ 8 pieces of smoked salmon meat or fresh organic salmon meat torn into smaller pieces.
- ❖ 4 avocados sliced into half
- ❖ 8 eggs
- ❖ Fresh rosemary and thyme
- ❖ Pinch of salt
- ❖ Olive oil

Directions:

1. Preheat the oven to 200 deg celsius
2. Scoop out the seed from each half of the avocado.
3. Arrange the avocados on a baking sheet on a baking tray.
4. Line the hole of the avocado halves with a slice of smoke salmon.
5. Carefully spoon the egg yolk and some egg whites to fill up the hole.
6. Sprinkle fresh herbs, rosemary and thyme on top with a pinch of salt and pepper.
7. Drizzle olive or avocado oil on top of the avocado halves.
8. Bake for 15 min until the eggs are soft but not over cooked.
9. Serve warm and enjoy!

Recipe 3) Golden Turmeric Tofu for Added Phytoestrogens During Menopause

Get good, clean, organic, non GMO tofu for this recipe which is a helpful dish to have during menopause as tofu is high in phytoestrogen and reduces the effects of low estrogen associated with menopause mainly hot flushes, dryness, mood swings etc. The added turmeric and spices provide antioxidants to help reduce inflammation associated with estrogen deficiency.

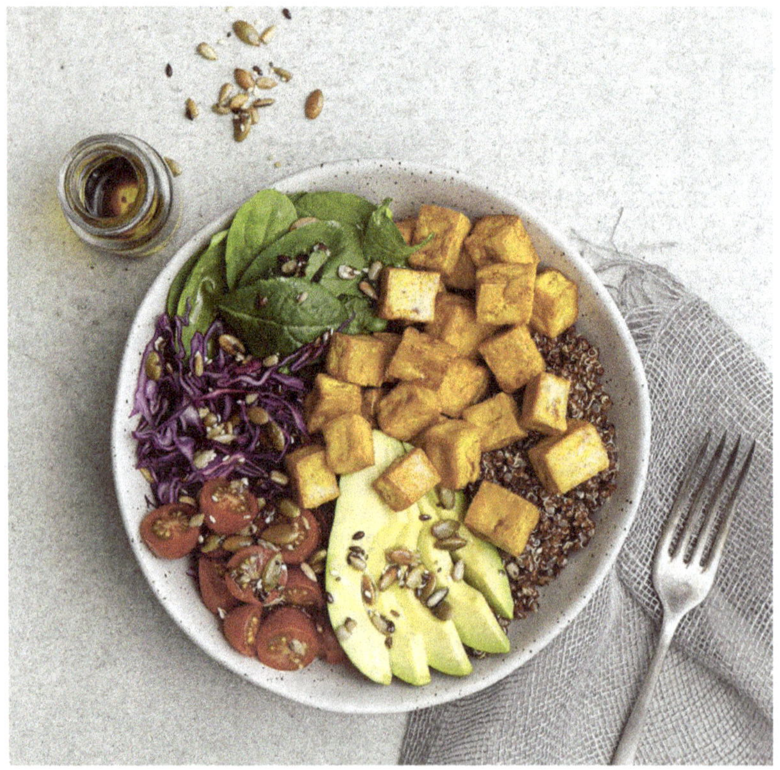

Serving: 4
Prep time: 10 min
Cooking time: 5 min

Ingredients:

- ❖ 300gm organic non GMO tofu
- ❖ Olive, avocado oil or rice bran oil
- ❖ 2-3 cloves of garlic finely diced
- ❖ Finely chopped ginger
- ❖ Finely chopped lemongrass
- ❖ Finely diced onions
- ❖ Spice mix : ½ tsp turmeric powder, ½ tsp herbal mix powder, ½ tsp cumin powder
- ❖ Pinch of salt

Directions:

1. Wrap the firm tofu with paper towels and squeeze out the excess water from the tofu to dry it.
2. Coat the tofu with the spice mix above evenly. You can choose to cut the tofu into smaller edible size pieces or leave it as a big piece of tofu.
3. To a medium heat non-stick frying pan, drizzle some olive oil and saute the onions, garlic and lemongrass until brown.
4. Add the pieces of tofu and cook over medium heat until one side is slightly brown. Turn to the other side and cook until the other side is slightly brown.
5. Season with a pinch of salt and a squeeze of lime.
6. Serve with some cabbage salad on the side with thai lime and vinegar dressing

Recipe 4) Fermented natto soybeans with avocado and egg rice bowl

Natto is a Japanese staple food made of soybeans that have been fermented for 24-36 hours to create a bacteria called bacillus subtilis. The soybeans are good as a source of phytoestrogen and the fermentation produces a natural probiotic which is also good for gut health. Pair this with avocado for good clean fats and top off with a poached egg makes this a wonderful and quick dish to have for breakfast or lunch. The topping of the seaweed provides additional iodine good for boosting thyroid function and the sesame seeds provides linoleic acid which is a natural source of phytoestrogens.

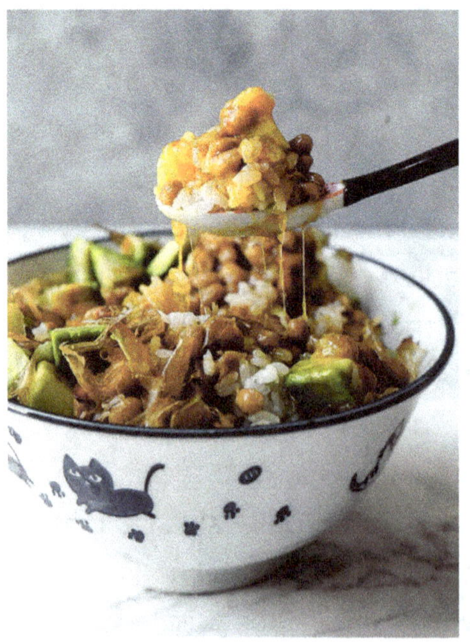

Serving: 1 bowl
Prep time: 10 min
Cooking time: 5min

Ingredients:

- 1 package natto
- 1/2 cup warm, cooked brown rice or Japanese short grain rice
- 1/2 avocado, chopped
- 1/2 cup English cucumber, seeded and diced
- 1 scallion, finely chopped
- Raw or poached egg
- Soy sauce for drizzling
- Bonito flakes or seaweed flakes
- Sesame seeds

Instructions

1. Cook the rice in a rice cooker. When cooked, place in a bowl.
2. Top with the natto, avocado and cucumber pieces.
3. Put the raw / poached egg on top of the ingredients.
4. Drizzle soy sauce over.
5. Sprinkle with bonito flakes or seaweed flakes.
6. Add the sesame seeds on top.
7. Enjoy!

Recipe 5) Green Detox Juice

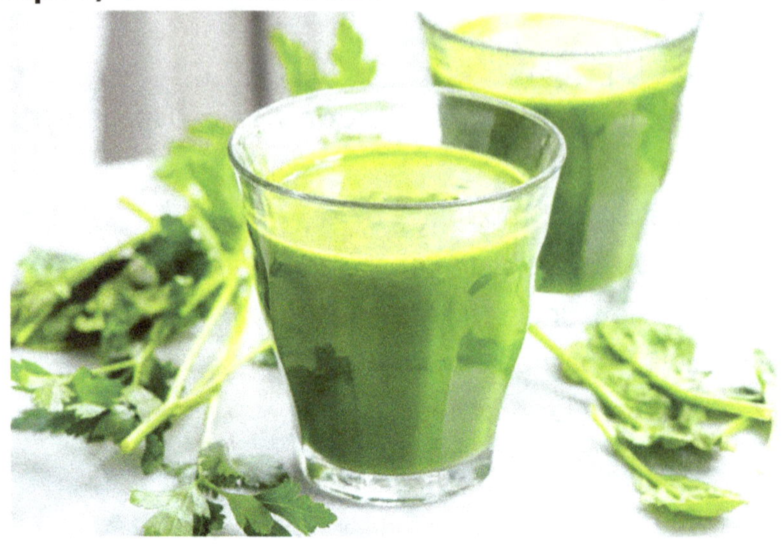

Benefits of the ingredients added into the juice

- Green apples are lower in sugar but still provide some sweetness to the juice. It is a good source of Vitamin A, C and potassium.
- Parsley or Cilantro is added as they are natural binders for toxins. They are high in antioxidants and rich in vitamins A, B, C, E and K and minerals like potassium, iron and magnesium.
- Spinach is easily added as it is light in taste but a good source of iron and is very alkalinizing which is good for detoxing.
- Cucumber and celery provide a good base for juices as it is a mineral rich water and provides a good source of vitamin A, B, C and folic acid.

- Lemons are good for balancing out the bitter taste. They are high in Vitamin C and antioxidants and are very alkalinizing which is good for detox.
- Ginger is anti-inflammatory and aids in digestion and reduces bloating. It is also warming to the body.

Ingredients:

- ❖ 2 cucumbers
- ❖ handful parsley
- ❖ handful mint
- ❖ 4 leaves spinach
- ❖ 5 stalks celery
- ❖ 2 cm piece fresh ginger, peeled if required
- ❖ 2 lemons, juice
- ❖ 1 green apple

Directions:

1. Juice all ingredients except lemon, pour into a glass and mix in lemon juice

Recipe 6) Alkalinizing and mineral rich vegetable broth

Servings: 8-10
Prep time: 15min
Cooking time: 1hr

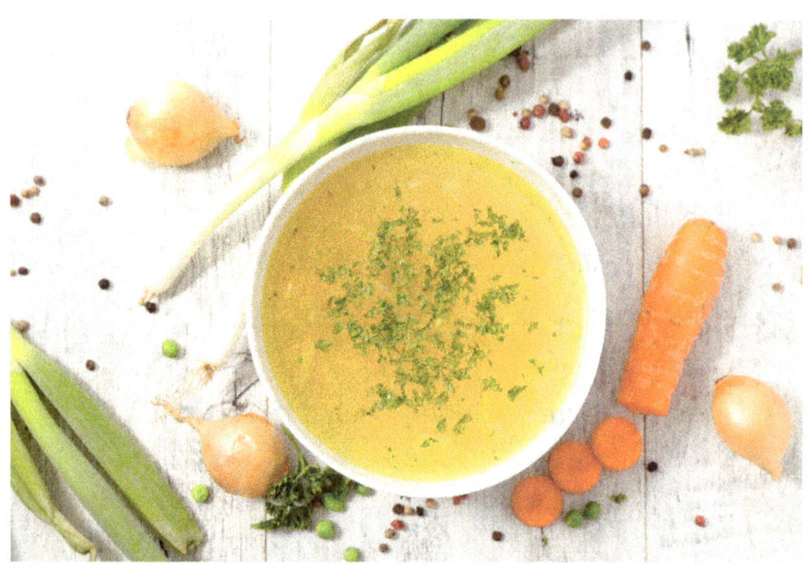

Ingredients:

- ❖ 2 onions chopped
- ❖ 4 medium size carrots
- ❖ 4 celery stalks, roughly chopped
- ❖ A bunch of parsley
- ❖ 2 Bay leaves
- ❖ Some dry herbs like oregano, thyme
- ❖ 1 tsp peppercorns (optional)
- ❖ Few pieces of ginger

Directions:

1. In a large pot, add some olive oil and sweat the onions until translucent and ginger pieces.
2. Add all other ingredients into the pot.
3. Cover with water about 1L (goes up to ¾ of the pot).
4. Place over high heat and bring to a boil, then reduce the heat and simmer for an hour with the lid half ajar. Stir the stock occasionally.
5. After an hour, taste the soup and add salt accordingly according to the taste.
6. When the stock is ready, turn off the fire and let it cool.
7. Once cooled, strain the soup into a colander to remove the herbs and vegetables and discard them.
8. Divide the stock into the storage containers for future use. Refrigerate for up to 4 days. If kept in the freezer can keep up to 3 months.

Recipe 7) Thai beef salad with kaffir lime and olive oil, peanut dressing

The beef in this salad provides adequate proteins and B vitamins which is helpful for strengthening the adrenals. Roast pumpkin is a good source of beta carotene and is a good source of resistance carbs that stabilizes the sugar and reduces mood swings and improves sleep. For hormones, we want more good fats in the diet which in this salad is provided by the olive and sesame oil and the nuts in the dressing. The turmeric and herb mix helps provide antioxidants and reduce inflammation.

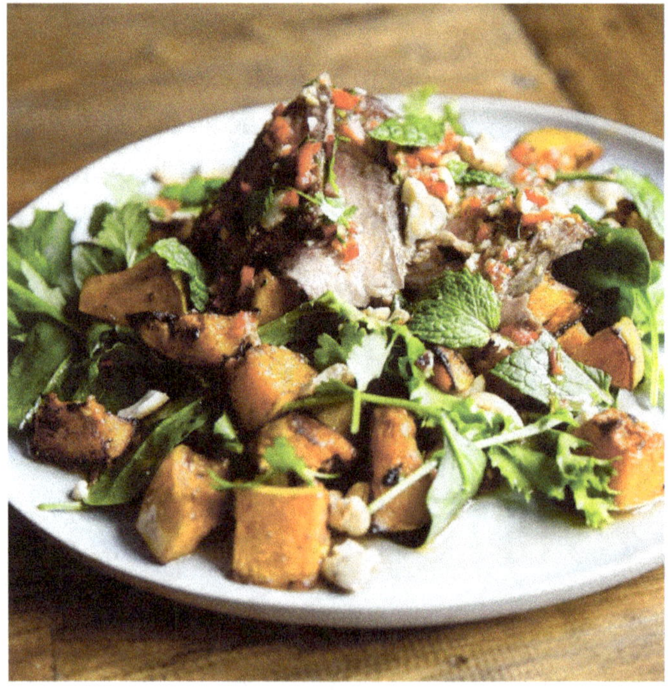

Servings: 2
Prep time: 15min
Cook time: 30min

Ingredients:

For the roasted pumpkin:
- ❖ 500gm pumpkin cut into 2-3 cm cubes
- ❖ Dry herb mix
- ❖ 1 tsp turmeric powder
- ❖ 1 tbsp olive oil
- ❖ Pinch of salt

Dressing:
- ❖ 1 stalk lemongrass, finely chopped
- ❖ 1 lime freshly squeezed for the juice
- ❖ Some finely chopped chillis
- ❖ Some grated ginger
- ❖ 2 cloves garlic finely chopped
- ❖ 2 tsp fish sauce
- ❖ 1 tbsp olive oil
- ❖ Drizzle of sesame oil
- ❖ Some sweet Thai chili sauce (optional)

Beef salad:
- ❖ 300gm organic grass fed beef filet
- ❖ 1 tsp spice mix
- ❖ Spinach or baby lettuce salad leave

Toppings:
- ❖ 1 tsp sesame seeds
- ❖ ¼ cup chopped almond nuts
- ❖ ½ thai mint and basil leaves chopped

Directions:

1. Preheat the oven to 200 deg celsius.
2. Line the baking tray with baking paper and put the cube pieces of pumpkin spread out on the tray and mix well with the dry herb mix and turmeric powder. Drizzle over the olive oil until the cubes are fully covered by the oil. Sprinkle with a pinch of salt.
3. Roast for 30 min until the pumpkin is slightly brown and caramelized.
4. Mix all the ingredients for the dressing and set aside.
5. For the beef filet, pat the filet dry with some paper towels. Rub the beef with the spice mix and a pinch of pink salt. In a frying pan on medium heat, put in some olive oil and when it starts to get hot, cook the steak on each side for 2-3 min each side until slightly brown but still soft on the inside. Do not overcook the beef. Let it rest and cool on the side for 5-10 min. Once cooled, slice the beef filet thinly to your liking.
6. In a mixing bowl, mix the salad leaves, the dressing sauce and the roasted pumpkin until well mixed. Divide these into individual serving bowls. Top it with the slices of beef.
7. Garnish with the thai basil and mint leaves and sprinkle sesame seeds on top.

Recipe 8) Hormone and liver supporting Arugula salad with chickpeas, avocado and rosemary tahini sauce.

This is a great salad perfect for balancing the hormones as it contains good fats from olive oil, the nuts and the avocado. The arugula leaves have benefits for enhancing liver detoxification. The herbs like rosemary and thyme provide antioxidants for boosting liver health and detoxifying excess estrogen. Chickpeas and quinoa provide good resistant carbs of stabilizing sugars and balancing the cortisol.

Servings: 1
Prep time: 10min
Cooking time: 5min

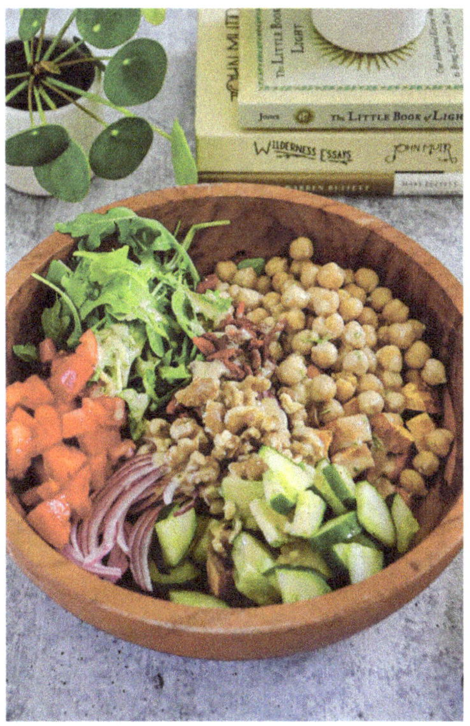

Ingredients:

- ❖ A handful of arugula leaves
- ❖ 1 cup of rinsed chickpeas
- ❖ 1 cup of cherry tomatoes
- ❖ ½ purple onion thinly sliced
- ❖ ½ avocado deseeded and cut into cubes
- ❖ ½ cup chopped almonds or walnuts and pumpkin seeds
- ❖ ½ chopped cucumbers
- ❖ 1 hard boiled egg (sliced)
- ❖ 1/2 cup quinoa

How to cook the quinoa

To ½ the cup of quinoa, add in 1 cup of water and cook uncovered until the quinoa has absorbed all the water. Remove the pot from the stove and leave the pot covered to steam the remaining quinoa for 5min. The quinoa will pop open and be perfectly cooked.

Dressing ingredient

- ❖ 2 tbsp tahini sauce
- ❖ Pinch of sea salt
- ❖ ½ tsp dried oregano
- ❖ ½ tsp dried thyme
- ❖ 1 tsp dried or freshly chopped rosemary
- ❖ 1 tbsp olive oil

Directions

1. In a small bowl, mix all the ingredients for the dressing.
2. In a salad bowl, add in all the ingredients for the salad - the arugula leaves, chickpeas, onions, tomatoes, avocados, cucumbers.
3. Mix in the quinoa.
4. Pour in the dressing and mix the salad well.
5. Enjoy!

Recipe 9) Korean Kimchi soup with beef, tofu and mushrooms

Kimchi is a great source of fermented cabbage which is rich in probiotics for maintaining good gut health. Organic, non GMO tofu provides phytoestrogens good for post menopausal ladies. Adding in sesame oil which is a source of lignans also acts on the estrogen receptors to help menopausal symptoms. Beef adds an added source of B vitamins and protein to the soup. But this is optional and can be taken out for a vegetarian version. Mushrooms add additional fiber and helps in boosting the immune system.

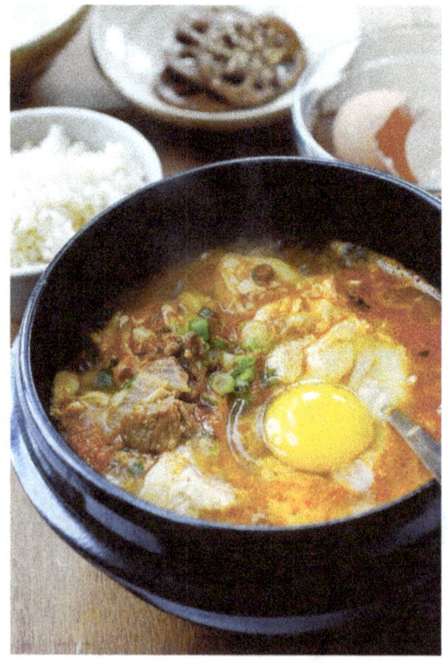

Servings: 2
Prep time: 15min
Cooking time: 15 min

Ingredients:

- ❖ 1 pack non GMO silken tofu
- ❖ ½ cup sliced fermented kimchi
- ❖ 100gm beef slices
- ❖ 1-2 tsp korean chili pepper flakes (according to spice tolerance)
- ❖ 2 cloves chopped garlic
- ❖ 1 tbsp sesame oil
- ❖ 500ml organic chicken broth
- ❖ 2-3 tbsp from Kimchi juice
- ❖ Pinch of salt
- ❖ Few stalk scallions, chopped
- ❖ 1 egg (optional)
- ❖ 1 pack of enoki mushroom

Directions:

1. In a small pot bring it to medium heat and lightly stir fry for about 3-4 min the chopped garlic with the beef slices in the sesame oil until lightly brown.
2. Add in the chopped kimchi and the chili flakes.
3. Add in the chicken broth, the kimchi juice and bring to boil for about 3-4 min, then lightly simmer on low heat for about 5 min.
4. Add in the silken tofu and enoki mushrooms and simmer for another 5 min.

5. Add a pinch of salt and pepper according to taste. Some store bought kimchi may be salty enough and hence you can omit the salt.
6. Top with the raw egg and sprinkle on the scallions. Take the pot off the fire.
7. Drizzle some sesame oil on top.
8. Serve and enjoy with some brown rice.

Recipe 10) Protein and Antioxidant Rich Edamame and Bibimbap Buddha Bowl

The Korean bibimbap is known for being a dish full of colorful vegetables and yet is delicious due to the Korean gochujang (Fermented soybean) sauce. In this version, I have made this into a vegetarian version with the main protein source not from the meat but instead from edamame beans, mushrooms and an optional egg.

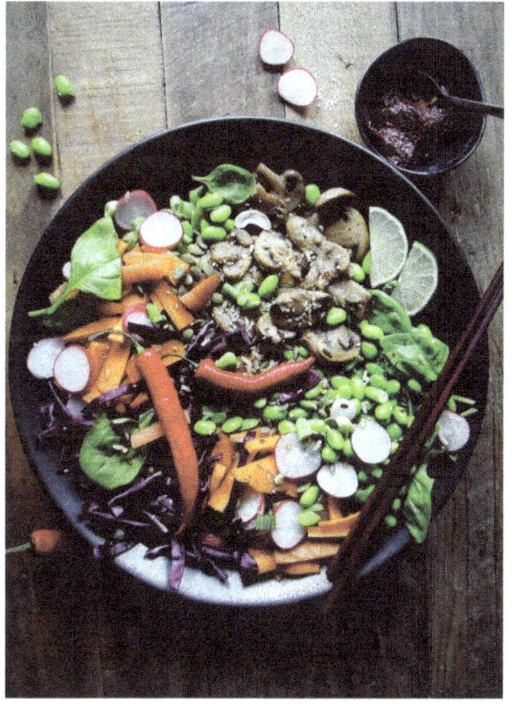

Servings: 2
Prep time: 15 min
Cook time: 30 min

Ingredients

For Bibimbap sauce:
- ½ cup gochujang (korean fermented chili paste)
- ¼ cup sesame oil
- 1/4 cup organic honey
- ¼ cup water
- ¼ cup toasted sesame seeds
- 1 tbsp apple cider vinegar
- 2 cloves minced garlic

For Bibimbap
- 1 cup organic brown rice cooked
- 2 cups Shitake mushroom, soaked and sliced
- 2 carrots thinly sliced
- ½ cup organic radish thinly sliced
- 1 cup of cooked edamame beans
- 1 cup red cabbage
- 1 handful spinach
- ¼ purple onions thinly sliced
- Seeds: including sunflower seeds and sesame seeds
- Chili flakes (optional)
- Poached egg (optional)

Directions

1. To cook the rice, rinse the rice under water and add in the boiling water till it covers the rice and cook for 25-30 min.
2. Meanwhile, prepare the sauce by mixing all the ingredients together.
3. In a pan, stir fry the mushrooms in sesame oil until lightly soft and cooked.
4. Prepare all the chopped raw vegetables.
5. In a bibimbap or mixing bowl, add the rice and layer the different vegetables with the mushrooms and edamame beans in a neat and colorful manner.
6. Top with the optional poached egg.
7. Sprinkle on the seeds and scallions.
8. Add on the sauce and mix everything well together. Add a pinch of salt and pepper to taste.
9. Enjoy!

References:

(1) Henmi H, Endo T, Kitajima et al. "Effects of ascorbic acid supplementation on serum progesterone level in patients with a luteal phase defect." Fertility and sterility 80 (2) (2003): 459-61

(2) Westphal LM, Polan ML, Trant, AS. "Double blind, placebo-controlled study of Fertilityblend: a nutritional supplement for improving fertility in women." Clinical and Experimental Obstetrics and Gynecology 33(4) (2006): 205-8.

(3) Nagata C, Shimizu H, Takami R, et al. "Hot flushes and other menopausal symptoms in relation to soy product intake in Japanese women." Climacteric 2(1) (1999): 6-12

(4) Kotsopoulos J, Eliassen AH, Missmer SA, et al. "Relationship between caffeine intake and plasma sex hormone cincentrations in premenopausal and postmenopausal women." Cancer 115 (12) (2009): 2765-74.

(5) Auerbach L, Rakus J, Bauer C, et al. "Pomegranate seed oil in women with menopausal symptoms." Menopause 19 (4) (2012):426-32

(6) Shams T, Setia MS, Hemmings R, et al. Efficacy of black cohosh-containing preparations on menopausal symptoms: a meta-analysis. 2010

(7) Kazemi F, Masoumi SZ, Shayan A, Oshvandi K. The Effect of Evening Primrose Oil Capsule on Hot Flashes

and Night Sweats in Postmenopausal Women: A Single-Blind Randomized Controlled Trial.

(8) Kim SY, Seo SK, Choi YM, et al. Effects of red ginseng supplementation on menopausal symptoms and cardiovascular risk factors in postmenopausal women: a double-blind randomized controlled trial. Menopause. 2012;19(4):461-6.

(9) Nordio M, Proetti E. "The combined therapy with myo-inositol and D-chiro-inositol reduces the risk of metabolic disease in PCOS overweight patients compared to myo-inositol supplementation alone." European Review For Medical and Pharmacological Sciences 16(5)(2012):575-81.

(10) Westphal LM, Polan ML, Trant, AS. "Double-blind, placebo-controlled study of Fertilityblend: a nutritional supplement for improving fertility in women." Clinical and experimental Obstetrics and Gynecology 33(4)(2006):205-8.

(11) Henmi H, Endo T, Kitajima Y, et al. "Effects of ascorbic acid supplementation on serum progesterone levels in patients with a luteal phase defect." Fertility and Sterility 80(2)(2003): 459-61.

(12) Hackney AC, Hosick KP, Myer A, Rubin DA, Battaglini CL. Testosterone responses to intensive interval versus steady-state endurance exercise. J Endocrinol Invest. 2012 Dec;35(11):947-50.